Unleash ___
Nerve

Stimulate Your Vagal Tone and Activate Its Healing Power with Daily Exercises to overcome Anxiety, Depression, Inflammation, Autoimmunity, Brain Fog, and Gut Sensitivities.

Yumi Park

CONTENTS

CHAPTER 1

—·—

THE WHAT NERVE, NOW?

The vagus nerve. If that doesn't ring any bells for you, then you've come to the right place. Because, as we'll come to see, this nerve plays a fantastically huge role in many aspects of our physical health and a surprisingly powerful part of our emotional states. This book will discuss how and why the vagus nerve is vital. Perhaps most importantly, it will discuss how to use this understanding to harness its power to help those of us who feel the constant burden of depression and anxiety. But before we dive into all things vagus, let's take a minute to discuss these emotional afflictions that have come to cast their shadows over so many of us.

It is no secret that the incidents of depression, anxiety, and other related stressors on our emotional lives are affecting an ever-widening percentage of people in the 21st century than before. According to the latest numbers from the World Health Organization, in 2017, more than 264 million people suffered from depression worldwide. Approximately 800,000 of these people commit suicide every year, making it the second leading cause of death in individuals aged 15–29 years. It is the leading cause of disability in the United States among people aged 15-44 years and if you are a person who believes that, as Bob Dylan put it, "Money doesn't talk, it swears," here comes a big F-bomb (F stands for financial, of course): The U.S. economy in 2017 lost roughly $210.5 billion dollars through worktime losses directly traceable to depression (National Network of Depression Centers).

Symptoms of persistent anxiety have a large overlap with those of depression, which is to be expected, as the two are essentially different sides of the same coin. But there are a few new tell-tale signs that anxiety brings to the table. They include trouble controlling one's breathing, feelings of nausea, increased irritability, sweating, heart palpitations, and, perhaps worst of all, a general and often untraceable but bone-deep feeling of dread and despair.

We are citing all of this not to make you feel hopeless; it is our hope that if you struggle with depression or anxiety, talking frankly at the outset about what's been happening to an increasing number of us over the last few decades will make you feel better. Even if you're not more comfortable with your depression/anxiety, you should feel more comfortable with the fact you are struggling because the numbers of individuals who are suffering like you are legion.

Here's a little more news that shines a light or perhaps more aptly casts a deeper shadow on the above information. Unsurprisingly, the emergence of the COVID-19 pandemic has only increased these numbers. According to the CDC:

"Between August 2020 and February 2021, the percentage of adults with recent symptoms of anxiety or a depressive disorder increased from 36.4% to 41.5%, and the percentage of those reporting an unmet mental health care need increased from 9.2%

to 11.7%. Increases were largest among adults aged 18–29 years and those with less than a high school education."

With much of the world closing restaurants, bars, cinemas, theaters, sporting arenas, cafes, and parks and moving schools to remote learning, thousands of businesses drowned in the treacherous economic waters roiled by the coronavirus, and most people were forced to shelter in place for months at a time. Because of this, it makes complete sense that the rates of mental health crises would skyrocket. This is to say nothing of the punishing and inhumane pressures, traumas, and hours first responders such as EMTs, nurses, and doctors had to endure, which led more than a few otherwise mentally stable medical professionals to resign due to profound trauma. Some of these workers were so emotionally savaged by the pandemic they even resorted to suicide.

The CDC goes further, stating, "Limits on operating nonessential businesses and other measures to reduce pandemic-related mortality led to isolation and unemployment or underemployment, further increasing the risk for mental health problems". Frankly, it will be years before we as a society will be able to accurately process and assess the amount and depth of scars that the worldwide COVID-19 crisis wrought on populations as a whole. This is even worse for children and young adults whose childhoods and young adulthoods were robbed of many of the normal interactions and rites of passage most mental health experts consider an essential part of emotional development.

Now, I know that this is not the most cheerful way to start a book, even if this book is about giving you real ideas and techniques that will help you to better cope with depression and anxiety. Also, we just threw a lot of numbers your way, which is usually not the punchy opening readers want as they crack open a new book. And what does all of this depressing news have to do with the vagus nerve? I mean, that is pretty much why you bought this book, isn't it? Let's get vagusing, you might well be saying.

I promise that I'll soon get to that without much further ado. But first, we need to know about what we're trying to battle against and how and why a growing number of experts believe the vagus nerve is one of our best hopes for coping with and even overcoming these dark feelings that so many of us are going through.

Yes, I will use more statistics to be sure but not at anything like this early rate. I feel it is important to provide some context for the problems we are dealing with. Understanding how the vagus nerve has an effect on all of this is important. Most of all, I want you to understand these numbers to put into perspective that you are not alone in your suffering or the suffering of one of your loved ones.

This is a book that will rely heavily on hard science but not written in jargon. As such, I should be precise where I can. I just rattled off some pretty grim statistics about depression, both in the United States and around the world. But, not to be too simplistic, let's start off by clarifying our terms, namely, what, exactly, according to medical authorities, constitutes depression? It's a word people like to throw around but how is it classified by the experts in mental health?

Doctors define depression as a syndrome. To better understand this, we should first define the word "syndrome." A syndrome, medically speaking, is not one basic attribute, but rather an amalgam of attributes, like bipolar and recurrent or monopolar depressive disorder. These are diagnosed when a patient presents with diminished or non-existent interest or pleasure in activities, which, as a direct result, makes it anywhere from very difficult to impossible to participate in the activities that make up everyday life.

There are other symptoms that branch out from this, including irregular sleep patterns (insomnia or its exact opposite, hyposomnia), loss of appetite or increase in appetite, impairment of cognitive functions, and a formless but palpable feeling of guilt.

There are many factors involved and the predominant agents of these troubling feelings and thoughts vary to one degree or another from individual to individual. Yet, for all of the miracles of modern science and medicine that we are blessed to have at our disposal, one area that has been relatively lacking is our knowledge of the workings of the brain, or more accurately, the mind.

However, we are quickly catching up and there is no shortage of positive news in this field. Researchers are steadily closing the knowledge gap and have made great progress in learning how our minds operate in just the last few decades; our collective understanding of the physiological operations regulating our emotional lives expands each year.

Anyone who has suffered from severe and persistent depression and/or anxiety is probably aware that there is no shortage of treatments. Many more are developed all the time. Medication has been a mainstay in such treatment for decades but the variety of medications available now is staggering. The specificity with which they target certain areas of the brain can sometimes yield promising results. In addition, there are many other options, such as transcranial magnetic therapy, ketamine, and even electroconvulsive therapy, known more commonly as electroshock. The latter has made a comeback in a far safer and more effective way than the type that was so calamitously employed in the early 20th century.

For all of these treatments and discoveries, perhaps one of the most significant is the discovery of the crucial role the vagus nerve plays in affecting our state of mind. As we will come to see, it's a stunningly important component of our mental health, which is vital in fighting depression and anxiety and reducing stress. So, it's perfectly natural to ask yourself the question, "What on earth is the vagus nerve, and why, if it's so important, haven't I heard of it?"

It's a fair point. After all, many of you could name at least a few antidepressants off the top of your heads, not to mention other treatments. If it is so crucial to our mental wellbeing (and the science consistently bears out that it is) then why isn't the vagus nerve more widely discussed? In truth, it is starting to gain a foothold in the public consciousness but we as a society need to become more aware of the myriad ways it is deeply involved with both our physical and emotional wellbeing.

This is one of this book's key aims. Another is to assist you in your fight against depression and/or anxiety by offering concrete advice on how to help you access the tremendous power of the vagus nerve to help you push back hard against these sometimes debilitating conditions. The possibilities for physical and emotional improvement by learning about and attending to the vagus nerve are real and quite profound. So, are you ready to learn about your relationship with this vital part of your body? Great! Let's start off, as any good relationship should, with a proper introduction.

The vagus nerve, like virtually every nerve in the human body, starts in the brain. Technically, it's actually two nerves that branch off from a single course. For the purposes of our discussion, we will generally be referring to them as one. And while the vagus nerve is only one of twelve cranial nerves, "this particular nerve is unique because it is associated with both sensory and motor functions".

The vagus nerve was first discovered relatively recently in terms of medicine. It was discovered about a hundred years ago, in 1921, by a doctor named Otto Lowei. It was shortly thereafter discovered as the first neurotransmitter, which is defined by Webster as a "chemical substance that is released at the end of a nerve fiber by the arrival of a nerve impulse and by diffusing across the synapse or junction." In plain language, it means that it releases a chemical that can send information to your brain by going through long channels and branches of subsidiary nerves.

The fact that the vagus nerve plays a central role in regulating our emotions didn't enter into the mainstream of scientific thought until 1988, which is more recent still. Given this, the amount of progress that has been made since is beyond impressive.

Stimulation of the vagal nerve decelerates the heart rate due to the release of acetylcholine (ACh). And while this information isn't important to know (if there were a quiz at the end of this book you wouldn't be required to remember it) the vagus became the first neurotransmitter ever discovered. However, this is partially why, unlike many other nerves (fun fact: our bodies have approximately 100 billion of them), which focus on a single area of the body, the vagus nerve is linked to many parts of our anatomy. In fact, it derives its name from the Latin word that means "to wander." It's an apt moniker. It is the longest nerve in the human body (another fun fact: if nothing else, our book has already helped you become the hit of any boring party) and is connected to a staggering number of organs, such as your liver, spleen, kidneys, pancreas, digestive system, lungs, heart, and beyond. Most critically for the purposes of our discussion, it plays a major role in regulating what is known as the "parasympathetic nervous system."

A quick word about that term you just read. This is a book that involves explaining an important scientific discovery, but it is absolutely not a science textbook. So don't be worried that you need a medical license to follow what we'll be delving into. Anything that may sound too technical, we will explain in plain language. There will be no pop quizzes or final exams.

Ok then, back to the parasympathetic nervous system. Its main responsibilities are the regulation of your digestion and rest. More broadly, it is a bit like your nervous system's behind-the-scenes movie director that makes sure that your body's various systems are working in harmony with each other. It plays a large part in helping our bodies recuperate from injuries and disease. It also has a heavy to-do list involving many other functions, including your body's involuntary or autonomic function or the things you do without giving them any thought but without which, you'd die. These include breathing, heartbeat, and your circulatory system.

It also involves vital functions such as speech, breathing, swallowing, libido, and taste. It even tells you when you need to pee. And what oversees this vastly important system? Our friend, the vagus nerve does. Therefore, the vagus nerve is indispensable for many of our most important anatomical processes. It also plays a critical role on our moods and sense of well-being.

For example, it notes when you've expended or are expending a great deal of energy (as shown by your heart rate) and ensures that your body will be primed for rest. It is able to prepare you more easily for rest by a variety of means, such as slowing your digestion and lowering your blood pressure. Have you ever wondered why, after a day of strenuous labor, you often feel exhausted? Of course you haven't; it's the most natural and logical thing in the world. No argument here; however, it is the Vagus nerve that largely creates that feeling. It is essentially ordering your body to get some rest.

Studies show that something on the order of 80% of the information transmitted by the vagus nerve goes from the body to the brain, which means that the brain transmits about 20% of the signals to the vagus nerve. This is perhaps why many scientists refer to the vagus nerve as our body's "second brain." In other words, the vagus nerve seems to literally have a mind of its own.

However, the vagus nerve is, so to speak, only human. If you find yourself under persistent stress and tension, which is a state that millions of us find ourselves in when navigating our daily lives, the vagus nerve itself doesn't get much of a breather. In fact, constant stress makes it overwhelmed. It then calls in what doctors call the sympathetic nervous system (this is in charge of what is commonly known as the "fight or flight" mode that your body switches on during stressful moments).

The vagus nerve seems to be a biological genius and it is. However, it is not immune to making the occasional error. When you feel overwhelmed, like when you have to make a presentation at work or have to endure a family gathering in which your uncle will explain his eccentric political beliefs in maddening detail, your vagus nerve is in the thick of it.

However, if that nerve is in some way damaged (and many of ours are to some degree, for a multitude of potential reasons that we will get into more specifically later), it often misinterprets your garden variety nervousness or discomfort for legitimate danger and activates the sympathetic nervous system.

When the vagus nerve isn't functioning properly, the sympathetic nervous system can sometimes lose perspective, which often results in high levels of anxiety and even outright panic attacks. It can act like the anatomical equivalent of calling in a military airstrike over a parking ticket and it takes a real toll on our emotional experiences. This is why when we're anxious, we often experience unpleasant physical symptoms such as sweating, an accelerated heartbeat, nausea, and so on.

If you've ever experienced these bodily symptoms under duress, it likely means that your vagus nerve is not functioning as it should. Welcome to the club! The vagus nerve is making your body react with too much anxiety to minor situations. As many of us have experienced, our tendency towards anxiety can reach a point in which that feeling lacks any conscious cause; it instead can feel at times like a persistent and sometimes maddening buzz that we can hear all the time. No matter how hard we try, we cannot locate its source. So, if you're feeling stress, depression, or anxiety, we can assure you that your vagus nerve is, too. In fact, it may well be a large part of the reason why you're feeling such emotional and mental distress. And even if it is not the primary cause, if your vagus nerve feels this way, it exacerbates your feelings in a deeply unpleasant reciprocal loop.

So, what happens when our vagus nerves are damaged? Well, to put it simply, a lot of things and none of them are pleasant. Among other issues, a damaged vagus nerve can result in such emotional and physical disorders as depression, anxiety, insomnia, obesity, circulatory issues, and even, in extreme cases, Parkinson's disease. The bad news, as you now know, is that many of us have damaged our vagus nerves to one degree or another. However, there is good news as well. This book is here to assure you that you have the ability to ensure that things will get better! I can work on helping your vagus nerve to heal, and through that healing, make yourself healthier both physically and emotionally.

So why do most of us have some sort of damage to our vagus nerves? Well, there are many reasons this could be the case and for a lot of people in modern society, there are often several reasons. If you suffer from chronic diseases, such as Parkinson's disease (which, paradoxically, as we just noted, can often lead to nerve damage), Huntington's disease, or diabetes, this will often cause nerves to not function properly. And here's a cruel irony about that: type two diabetes can be brought on by factors such as obesity and lack of physical activity. A damaged vagus nerve can also lead to either rapid and unhealthy weight loss or, conversely, obesity. As we've covered in some detail already, depression, which often results in a marked lack of physical activity can also be a contributing factor.

Likewise, bodily trauma, such as a car accident, can jostle the nerve slightly out of alignment. For that matter, so can any jolting injury, like playing football, a particularly enthusiastic romp in a mosh pit in the 90s, or a hockey collision. Sometimes, the injury's cause may even occur accidentally during the course of surgery. Remember, this is the longest nerve in the body, starting at the medulla, which is located in the back of the brain, and going all the way down to the colon. In addition, it has a vast amount of subsidiary channels that go to virtually every organ in our bodies. Given all of these factors, any injury involving a collision makes the vagus nerve a prime candidate for injury.

Smoking and heavy drinking can also cause damage to the nerve. The same applies to a poor diet that relies on too much sugar, salt, and junk food. This makes sense, of course, as the nerve plays such a vital part in our digestive system.

This means that damage to the nerve will often result in digestive complications such as gastroparesis, a less than enjoyable condition whose symptoms can include severe and persistent bouts of nausea and heartburn. This is only a small list of issues that can happen with a less than operational vagus nerve.

By now, I think we're all on the same page (literally) about the vital nature of the vagus nerve. We've talked about what makes it important. Now let's look briefly into how it plays such important and multi-varied roles. When discussing the vagus nerve, medical experts generally divide its functions into four broad categories. The first involves the sensory functions of our bodies. These processes are in turn subdivided into two distinct types of sensory activities. What's known as the "somatic component" is in charge of your skin's ability to feel and swallow. Believe it or not, despite how naturally most of us do it, swallowing is, anatomically, a highly complex activity.

In fact, many victims of a stroke that affects the vagus nerve also need prolonged and difficult physical therapy with speech pathologists to relearn that skill. It involves three separate muscles and it must be regulated to make sure you are able to maintain a regular breathing pattern. It also makes sure that whatever you're eating is blocked from entering your airway passages. If you've ever had the unpleasant experience of food going down the "wrong pipe," you know how important this act is.

The next category is the motor, which involves dealing with much involuntary movements, such as heartbeat and breathing. It also oversees our digestive process. When food enters your stomach, the vagus nerve dispatches the various acids the stomach needs to break the food down into its nutritional components as well as wipe out unhealthy bacteria. Another important component is the special sensory system, which assists in our ability to taste.

CHAPTER 2

— · —

TRUST YOUR GUT

Because the vagus nerve plays such an important role in both heartbeat and breathing, when we experience stress and anxiety, taking slow deep breaths can often reduce the level of those negative experiences. When we experience stress or anxiety, the vagus nerve's response is to speed up both the rate of breath and the heartbeat (in order to fight or flee). Deliberately slowing down one's breathing sends a message, if you will, that things are under control, and therefore the nerve sends the signal to lower the heartbeat as well as accommodate slower breathing (which is why after the first few breaths, slow breathing often becomes easier). Again, we can see in this example how our emotional experiences and the reaction of our vagus nerves are intimately linked and one is constantly informing the other.

As the vagus nerve plays such a large role in our digestive system, you might conclude that it also plays a role in regulating our feelings of hunger (or lack thereof). And you'd be right. If a vagus nerve is functioning less than optimally, it can fail to send our brains the signal that we feel sated. Again, this is a big part of why many of us eat more than we should when we feel depressed.

Of course, there are often profound psychological factors at play as well but the vagus nerve's ability to mitigate those impulses is weakened. Alternatively, it may do the exact opposite and tell our brains we're full to the point where eating anything more is unthinkable to us, despite the fact we've actually eaten very little. This can lead to unhealthy rapid weight loss and severe malnutrition.

We've all had "butterflies" that we feel in our stomach when we are in the first throes of infatuation or that slight queasiness when we sense something unpleasant is heading our way. The expression "gut feeling" is in fact often quite literal. Scientists actually call this the gut-brain axis, which is mercifully an uncomplicated term. The vagus nerve is always on alert for changes in our emotional states, and it bases a lot of this observation on monitoring the gut.

This goes beyond merely telling our brains whether or not we need food, although that's a pretty important piece of information to have. This communication is what makes the vagus nerve inform our gut about how to feel. In many ways, it's best to understand the vagus nerve as the brain's ultimate intelligence gatherer, dictating to the brain how and where to best deploy its resources. This is why maintaining a healthy digestive system will, believe it or not, affect both your physical and emotional lives. How do we improve our gut health? There are many things we can do, including taking probiotic supplements and including foods rich in probiotics.

So, we've focused quite a bit on the problems that can arise from a damaged vagus nerve (and again, the term "damaged" isn't intended to induce panic). But let's not lose sight that there are several ways of repairing it. We'll explore these ways in more depth in future chapters, but we'll name a basic but important one here as a sort of appetizer, if you will. Some of you may not be thrilled to hear this, but there are few things more effective at this task than exercise.

Why? Because if you exercise with as much vigor as you can (and of course, it's important to discuss this with your doctor before embarking on any exercise regimen), the vagus nerve also exercises with you. When you've completed your exercise, you tend to feel happy and proud of your accomplishment. The vagus nerve then learns to associate this sort of activity, namely, pushing one's body to exert itself physically with positive feelings.

You've no doubt heard too many times to count that exercise is a terrific way of fighting depression, anxiety, and stress. It's true and the vagus nerve is a big part of the reason why. Plus, you'll be improving your body's overall health, which also helps the vagus nerve. In many cases, you're also improving your confidence, another mitigator of depression and anxiety. These are some of the ways that the vagus nerve has a profound physiological impact on our emotional lives.

Ideally, we want the vagus nerve to be highly responsive. The extent to which it is or it isn't the primary determinant of its health, which is something that doctors call the "vagal tone." Get used to that term; it will be coming up a lot. A low vagal tone is not good news. Research has shown again and again that a low vagal tone contributes to depression, anxiety, obesity, disruptive sleep patterns, persistent fatigue (which of course impedes both our reflexes and brain function), cardiovascular issues, and other things we don't want. It pretty much contributes to just about any negative physical, emotional, and even intellectual experience we can have other than a low credit score.

"Yikes," many of you must be thinking. Or maybe you just dropped another f-bomb. So, how do we measure vagal tone? It's not like there's a vagal tone monitor shop at a strip mall near you. Fortunately, there are ways you can still do it.

Ok, a quick trigger warning: we're about to throw a fancy-sounding medical term or two at you. However, we have a heart, so there is some good news: we're going to mostly refer to it as a three-letter abbreviation. So, the term we should understand that relates to vagal tone is "respiratory sinus arrhythmia," which would be great words in Scrabble, but not so fun to remember. We'll be referring to it from here on in as RSA. This condition is very common and largely pretty harmless. Basically, it's the normal variation in heart rate that occurs during each breathing cycle we discussed earlier. The heart rate increases when breathing in and decreases when breathing out.

A key sign is the variety of your heart rate, which means essentially to what degree do your heartbeats vary in their length between each other. Most of us think our heart rate is generally uniform, and it generally is in most people in reasonably good health. But it is seldom if ever exactly precise. The variation is usually a question of milliseconds. Incidentally, the normal heartbeat rate for most adults is somewhere between 60-100 beats per minute. Any heart rate that is above or below that is potentially problematic and if you fall into that category, it is important to consult with your medical professional.

And here's some even more, and even more fun facts (there's a point to all of this, we swear!): RSA tends to be higher when you're standing up and lower when you're lying down, which is pretty common-sensical when you think about it. Just as logically, it tends to be higher during the day than at night. Duh.

Most scientists believe that RSA probably evolved to conserve energy for both the heart and respiratory system when we perceive no danger. So, why does this matter? Because, while evolutionarily brilliant, we now have largely evolved as a culture in which confrontations with enemy tribes or grizzly bears have become relatively uncommon. And while for the most part, this is regarded as a good thing, it does mean that this capability sometimes has no use and can turn against us. This isn't to say we don't experience stress, in fact it can be argued that although we don't as a rule experience the life and death dangers that our ancient ancestors did, we may experience a far more consistent level of relatively low-grade stress with little respite. This may be why our vagus nerve, having nowhere to expend this energy in the short bursts it may have been evolved for, turns inward towards our minds, which may be a potent force in producing anxiety and depression.

Worse, for people like us, who aren't especially young (I mean, we're not ancient or anything. For example, we do have to occasionally ask for help when downloading apps, but we know precisely what both the words "downloading" and "apps" mean) are at an even greater disadvantage. As people age, the intensity of RSA tends to become less, although people in excellent physical health, especially athletes, tend to exhibit strong RSA levels well into old age.

There are ways of determining RSA numbers yourself, but you can also ask your doctor to help you. Your doctor will likely write you a note for a laboratory that specializes in such tests. This might sound intimidating. It can also feel intimidating when the technician attaches various electrodes to your body, but it's painless and accurate. The test is called an ECG. For those of you who may own watches that monitor your health constantly, however, there's more good news: many such watches have

ECG devices built-in and many have been given the FDA's seal of approval. So you can avoid those electrodes that are painless, but often involve a sticky, goopy substance that's annoyingly hard to scrub off in the shower.

Vagal tone research has the potential to offer insight into social behavior, social interactions, and human psychology. Much of this work has been focused on newborns and children. RSA and vagal tone are used as markers to help determine the severity of neurodevelopmental disorders such as autism spectrum disorders. Other studies have yielded more fascinating results. For example, children who enjoy more intimate and secure connections with their mothers exhibit greater empathetic responsiveness and greater self-confidence. In themselves, these results are hardly surprising. But guess what else kids also tend to almost universally have? I'm sure by this point, you've already guessed it: higher vagal tones.

Most scientists have grown confident about their assertions about our vagal tones as well as our understanding of exactly how and why they occur. This area of study is one of great interest and it's hard to believe our understanding of these details won't continue to grow at a quick rate in the next few years. What almost all researchers agree on is that an accurate reading of vagal tone opens a wide window into understanding its effects on social behavior, mental illness, and other aspects of psychology.

Moreover, the understanding of how and why vagal tone influences both the vagus nerve and our psychological states will likely give us greater insight into predicting what behavioral patterns are likely to emerge for people as they mature, which is why so much of the research has been directed at newborns and children. Though not conclusively proven yet, establishing a core vagal tone in young children can help predict how the children are likely to process the management of their emotions, anxiety, depression, and their general ability to manage their emotional lives.

Knowledge of RSA and vagal tone levels has started to be employed in some situations to assess the severity of neurological issues such as various autism spectrum disorders. We have spoken of the health of our vagus nerves as having a reciprocal relationship, a theory which is borne out with more potent evidence each year by these types of research.

By now I think we not only know that the vagus nerve is in many ways central to a seemingly endless array of vital functions of our mental and physical health, but we have a basic understanding as to why. As we've been hinting, you can even use these facts as an ice-breaker at dinner parties, though in all candor we wouldn't recommend it.

But we do think that our newfound knowledge can help us go a long way to improving our health by decreasing the likelihood and severity of obesity, cardiovascular disease, sleep disruptions, depression, anxiety, and deep-rooted as well as everyday stress. Now, let's get into a little more specific examples of how so many of our emotional responses to the world around us and within us are controlled by this nerve.

For most of us living in the 21st century, the stress in everyday life is quite simply unavoidable. In fact, there are evolutionary advantages to stress, even in our times. It can motivate us to finish that project we've been putting off rather than binge on a show on our favorite streaming platform, for example. But increasingly, modern society is often awash with stressors both large and small. Running late to pick up the kids, an unreasonable boss, an expensive repair to a car or home are all sources of stress. Even seemingly minor issues like, say, having to figure out a last-minute birthday present for your insufferable brother-in-law, causes a degree of stress. And then there are social media. Let's talk about this for a second.

Social media can be a tremendous source of stress for many people, especially teens and preteens. But it is hardly exclusive to that demographic. From futile yet blood boiling political debates with someone who you shared gym class within fourth grade to wondering where you went wrong while looking at your friends' pictures of bliss, harmony, and success (even their pets look happier than yours), your self-esteem is constantly eroded on these platforms. The irony is that social networks were ostensibly designed to build a sense of community, but instead they often leave us feeling alienated and isolated.

Let's not forget to take into account the severe trauma or even PTSD that many in modern society suffer from, whether it be from the loss of a loved one or a job, the enormous and sometimes overwhelming task of trying to make ends meet, or returning from the savagery of war. Modern life has no shortage of potential blows to mental health.

In short, modern life is often a minefield of small but relentless negative experiences. As a result, our vagus nerve calls out the battle-weary troops in the sympathetic nervous symptom to fend off this assault. But this too helps to create even more unease within our bodies. Oftentimes, these stress events happen so often that the vagus nerve never has a chance to do much other than try to hold on for dear life, so to speak. As is the case for most other animals, constant stress leads to a diminished capacity to function. In fact, the vagus nerve is often unable to stave off these issues, which is why we can lapse into chronic depression and anxiety or have feelings of failure.

An overwhelmed vagus nerve doesn't communicate nearly as well with the brain, which in turn causes the brain to produce an excess of chemicals that directly lead to feelings of depression and anxiety. These problems can in turn lead to obesity and even inflammation of organs and joints, which then makes our bodies vulnerable to a host of other diseases.

Let's talk a little bit about inflammation. Inflammation isn't always a bad thing; in fact, it's often a sign that your body is hard at work repairing an injury or fighting an infection. But even when it is happening for positive reasons, anyone who's ever experienced swelling, be it from an infection or a sprained ankle, will know that it doesn't feel good. So, what does the vagus nerve have to do with inflammation?

Well, the parasympathetic nervous system (the one that is in charge of handling our bodily actions that we are unaware of and have no conscious control of), under orders from your brain that are transmitted via the vagus nerve, kicks into action, expanding the blood vessels nearest to the infection site to release more antibodies and swelling injuries to help protect the injured area from further harm. Again, to use the same analogy as we employed in the previous pages of this book, it's easiest to think of the vagus nerve as a head coach or manager. Once it dispatches the parasympathetic nervous system to the problematic area, it feels confident that things are under control and it can tell the rest of the body that everything is being handled. Therefore raised heart rate lowers, breathing becomes fuller and less rapid, and a general sense of physiological and emotional calm can once again establish itself. That is, of course, if the vagus nerve is firing on all cylinders.

But when the nerve is less than at the top of its game, its ability to act swiftly and powerfully becomes diminished to the same degree that the nerve is unhealthy. An unhealthy vagus nerve can have trouble restoring a proper heart and breathing rate, putting a strain on both your body and your emotional state. It also becomes less effective at regulating the normally healthy reaction of swelling, allowing it to linger for an unnecessary length of time, and in some cases even become chronic.

Not only is such a condition, as you can no doubt imagine, both emotionally and physically painful, it can also open the door to painful chronic diseases such as lupus and arthritis. So, listing inflammation as a possible side effect of a damaged vagus nerve, when mentioned alongside such ailments as heart disease and circulatory disorders, might have sounded like a relatively minor affliction. However, it can have calamitous consequences. As we now can see, it is something to be avoided if at all possible. The odds of fending off inflammation decrease quite a bit if your vagus nerve isn't up to par.

As we mentioned, the increasing sense of isolation many of us feel in today's world is a widespread phenomenon. Those who have struggled with depression for any length of time will tell you that one of its primary effects is a profound need to withdraw from other people. They will also tell you that friends and therapists will argue quite correctly that social engagement with friends and family can reduce that sense of deep and abiding existential despair and sadness. Oftentimes, in fact, simply going out into public and having simple exposure to other people can improve one's mood.

Likewise, unfortunately, depression sufferers will also tell you that, while in the throes of clinical depression, going out and meeting people feels as difficult and overwhelming as running a marathon up a cliff. They simply cannot bring themselves to do it, even though they likely know it would help. Guess what helps to cause that feeling? You guessed correctly if you said the vagus nerve. Our vagal tone, absent during particularly stressful interactions, consistently improves in social settings, and suffers during periods of prolonged isolation. Your mileage may vary, in this respect. Introverts and extroverts require different levels of social engagement but all of them require them to some degree. So, what happens is a catch-22. The more depressed you become, the more isolated you become, which in turn hurts your vagal tone, which in turn makes you more prone to being depressed, which will invariably lead to more isolation, which then hurts your vagal tone even more, which…well, you get the idea.

Exercise, as we discussed earlier, is a wonderful way of improving our vagal tone and our physical health. But again, we face a cruel irony. For many of us, motivating ourselves to regularly exercise can be a struggle when we're feeling fine. Even people who enjoy being physically active find it exceptionally hard to muster up the mental energy to get off the couch when they're depressed. So when we don't move around a lot during the day, as many of us do, without exercise, we can often find it hard to sleep well. Our bodies still have energy to burn. Some people with serious depression react in the opposite manner, all they tend to do is sleep. Either way, it leads to the same problem. It throws our circadian rhythms, the part of the brain that regulates our sleep cycles, completely out of whack. Our obsession with screens, from tablets to televisions to phones doesn't help either, as the blue light which emanates from these electronic devices can sometimes trick the brain into believing it's still daylight.

Well, we all know what happens when we don't get enough sleep, right? We become less agile physically and mentally and forgetful. Chronic lack of sleep often lowers our defenses against illness. It also affects the vagus nerve's quality of communication with the brain, which in turn reduces the brain's capacity to produce chemicals like melatonin, which, ironically, is the chemical that enables us to sleep easily and soundly.

Boy, there has been a lot of distressing news in these last few pages. But do not despair! We would not have written this book if we didn't believe wholeheartedly that there are ways of reversing all of these trends that lead to physical and emotional challenges. In the chapters ahead, we'll explore specific steps that you can take to improve your vagal tone. There are steps all of us can do, and the science is now quite clear about the fact that improving our vagal tones will quite literally improve virtually every aspect of our lives.

CHAPTER 3

FREE GOODWILL

I hope you're enjoying the book so far and finding it helpful. Research has found that another way to help you feel better is to give to others. It's true. Donating to others fires off endorphins (the feel-good chemicals in our brains) like nobody's business and it will give you a justifiable sense of pride about making a difference in someone's life.

Here's my question to you: Would you want to make a positive difference in someone's life, a person you don't know and likely will never know if it cost you nothing but a minute out of your time?

I hope you said yes because I have a great and simple way for you to accomplish this: by leaving an honest review of this book. I believe strongly that this book can provide great help to the many who suffer from depression and anxiety. If you do, too, please leave an honest review of this book to help to spread the word.

All too often, people don't heed the classic warning about judging a book by its cover, as lovely as this cover may be. Your honest assessment of this book will have a strong influence on those contemplating whether or not it is right for them.

- You'll also be helping an entrepreneur to help build their business: a business grounded in trying to help others by making them aware of the role that the vagus nerve plays in their emotional health.

- Employees feel that they are doing meaningful work by learning techniques to improve their vagal tone.

- People will discover all the ways in which they can fight back against depression and anxiety by implementing what they learned here about the vagus nerve and how to keep it and themselves healthy and happy.

- Your review provides help for people who need it.

That's a lot of objectively great things to accomplish in 60 seconds.

Did I mention how it will give you a sense of wellbeing, too?

If you're the sort of person who's willing, or perhaps even eager, to make the world a little better, I thank you and I also think you're awesome. I think you'll find the chapters to come even more helpful in your own quest for a happier outlook on life.

And now, back to our regularly scheduled programming. Thanks, again!

Chapter 4

Let's Just Take a Breath, but the Right Kind of Breath

Okay: take a deep breath.

We aren't trying to be too critical. We're all on the same team here but the truth is that many of us just flat out don't breathe correctly. This may sound absurd. After all, we're getting our fair share of air, and isn't that the whole point of breathing? Well, as it turns out, not entirely. We used to breathe correctly. For example, as babies, we breathed beautifully, but then again, we had a lot less to get done back then. But for a host of reasons known and unknown, as we grow older, we start breathing incorrectly.

This raises a reasonable question: what do we mean when we claim that we breathe incorrectly? Put simply, we learned to breathe with the wrong parts of our body. Our breathing tends to be centered in the chest, as opposed to the diaphragm muscles in our abdomen; not only does this mean we are forced to include parts of our body that weren't designed with breathing in mind, but we don't breathe nearly as deeply. "Great," you may be thinking, "now I have to worry about how I breathe?" Well, the thing is, there's some very good news about this. It can be corrected over time. And why is this so important a thing to work on correcting? Because deep breathing is mother's milk to the vagus nerve; it's its happy place. This is another reason why consciously slowing our breathing and taking deep breaths are very good and simple techniques to feel a greater sense of calm.

In fact, let's delve into this point in a little more detail. Breathing deeply seems simple enough. We've done it for years when a doctor presses their inevitably ice-cold stethoscope on our backs and commands us to "take a deep breath," or when we blow out birthday candles. But while that's a good start, there's a little more to our definition of "deep breathing" than stuff like that. Deep breathing, if done correctly and practiced regularly, will have an effect on your mental state that will in all probability shock you.

So, how should you do it correctly? The key is breathing with your diaphragm, which will, at first, take some concentration and effort. It may sound easy, but many of us will find it hard. Some will find it very hard, at first. Here's what most experts agree is the best way to relearn this skill. You should first make yourself comfortable on the floor, or any reasonably solid even surface, with something to make your head comfortable, like a cushion, a pillow, or your trusted teddy bear, for that matter. We won't judge.

You should then place one hand on your chest and another on your stomach. The reason for this is simple: you will be able to feel the difference between breathing in a shallow manner and a deep one. A deep cleansing breath will cause your stomach to rise, as opposed to feeling a shallow breath gather in your chest.

Incidentally, a serious and devoted practice in this process is a given for any trained actor or vocalist. For one thing, it protects the larynx. Shallow breathing, if done throughout a long bout of vocalizing, will corrode the vocal quality to a quiet rasp, which, by the way, is your vocal chord's way of saying, "You're hurting me!" Done over time, it may lead to permanent damage. Secondly, it will give you far more control over your breath and make your voice far louder. Think about it, when we shout, most of us do it from our throats. But a truly booming voice can only come from the diaphragm.

Also, this may feel silly at first, but it's really important that you close your eyes when you're doing this. Why? There's not some strange medical reason for this involving another nerve you haven't heard of. It's simply because it will allow you to concentrate better on your breathing without distractions.

Some of you might find the transition fairly easy. That's great. But for most of us, at first, it requires a paradoxical mix of concentration and relaxation. Ideally, you want to perform these exercises daily each morning for at least five minutes. And when it's done correctly, you should be averaging roughly a half dozen breaths per minute. That sounds like very little, but this should give you a good sense of the deliberate and unhurried tempo you are aiming for. Some individuals will have to work harder than that, unfortunately. If you feel that you can only achieve deep breathing for one to three minutes or if you're breathing about ten times per minute, you're doing great! Like any other physical activity, you will improve with practice. Let's look at why this is the case.

Again, according to "Frontiers of Psychiatry" magazine in March of 2018, "breathing-based meditative technique stimulates the vagus nerve and exerts numerous autonomic effects, including changes in heart rate, improved cognition, and improved bowel function" You read that last part correctly. And while we assume no one wants us to dwell on this topic, let's be honest. Strong and regular bowel function is a healthy sign the body is working as it should.

Deep breathing calms the vagus nerve. It also provides a larger percentage of oxygen to your blood cells, which is a very good thing. Why? Because that allows the brain to produce and release endorphins more frequently and in greater volume. Endorphins are what make you feel happy. So, that is a very good thing.

By the way, as we've alluded to earlier, deep breathing shouldn't be restricted to a daily ritual. If you're having a moment of real stress during the day and feel your body about to be hit with a tidal wave of anxiety, deep breathing will, at minimum, greatly diminish the size and power of that wave. It seems almost too simple to be true, although learning to do it correctly on a consistent basis may very well take some time. But how can simply changing how we breathe mitigate our anxiety and depression? Well, don't forget that the human body, while not entirely perfect in design, is, when you're treating it right, a remarkable engine that is both complex and simple.

Trust us, deep breathing isn't the whole answer, but it's a big part of it.

One thing that you can do to improve your breathing is yoga. Multiple clinical studies have demonstrated the effectiveness of yoga as not only an excellent way of developing healthy breathing techniques, but also to mitigate the effects of depression and PTSD.

Here's another way to help your vagus nerve. And that's singing. You may not be the best singer in the world, but it's still worth a try. The Beatles may well have been onto a deep truth when they urged young Jude to "Take a sad song/ And make it better." Perhaps they had an unconscious sense that singing can play an important role in the readjusting of our vagus nerve.

Singing, preferably loudly, has a direct positive effect on the vagus nerve. Now, a lot of us aren't necessarily blessed with the best voices. We strongly urge you to get over it. Singing in the shower is always fun and the combination of rushing water and the acoustics of the tile is perfectly suited to make your voice reach its best. Drive a car? Well, that's not only a convenient mode of transportation, it is also the perfect stage for belting out along with your favorite songs. Join a choir, sing with friends around a fire, sing while you're vacuuming or mowing the lawn. If you're a musician, make it a point to play and sing every day when you get the chance. The clear, deep, and proven relationship between singing and improved mental health is directly related to the vagus nerve.

When you're singing, the vagus nerve assumes you're feeling safe and happy and therefore it quickly adjusts your body so it can relax. Furthermore, if you get past any self-consciousness you may initially feel, it's a lot of fun to sing along with your favorite artists or even sing your own tunes. This helps to create a positive feedback loop between you and your vagus nerve. Yes, feedback loops, discussed earlier because of their negative effects, can be a force for good!

In a similar way, many Eastern faiths and practices involve chanting, often involving prescribed traditional chants or prolonged humming. It's hard to believe the ancients who started these practices had any scientific data to support the importance of singing but they were no doubt deeply and correctly attuned to the connection between chanting and an improved and more peaceful state of mind. Westerners have sometimes unfortunately looked askance at such practices but it turns out we would all benefit from embracing these activities and their potential for healing and a greater sense of contentment.

If all of this perhaps sounds a little too unscientific, we get it. But, as we've shown you already, the scientific community is rapidly coming to understand the importance of the vagus nerve in managing our mental health. You don't have to take our word for it. But, we reckon, if you are the type who has a hard time picturing themselves sitting in a lotus position, greeting the day with gratitude, and communing with the Cosmos, it stands to reason that you would be more swayed by empirical, evidence-based information. Well, you've come to the right place.

We know that meditation and mindfulness can be great health tools, especially due to the positive effect they can have on the nervous system. Studies repeatedly and unambiguously show that practicing a type of meditation that focuses on self-care or what Buddhist monks have called "loving, kind meditation" not only improves vagus nerve tone, but also significantly reduces symptoms of depression in PTSD sufferers. It also helps to increase social connections. You may read this and find it somewhat self-indulgent, but it is an approach that quite simply is supported by Western scientific studies conducted by people who are most likely to be skeptical about anything related to crystals, tarot cards, or essential oils. If, however, you are open to this way of viewing the world, you probably won't need much convincing in the first place.

That cohort of researchers naturally inclined towards skepticism about meditation include doctors, like clinical psychologist Dr. Arielle Hausman, who has written, "By developing an understanding of the workings of your vagus nerve, you may find it possible to work with your nervous system rather than feel trapped when it works against you." Trust us, she is absolutely not an outlier among her colleagues. Dr. Mladen Golubic, the Medical Director of the esteemed Cleveland clinic, asserts with absolute confidence that "The vagal response reduces stress. It reduces our heart rate and blood pressure. It changes the function of certain parts of the brain, stimulates digestion, all those things that happen when we are relaxed." When it comes to humming and chanting as a salve for the vagus nerve, there's also no lack of scientific evidence. Dr. Stephen Porges conclusively showed that the vibrations these noises require from the larynx stimulate your vagus nerve quite quickly.

Given the nerve's intimate association with the larynx, this makes sense. If you don't believe us, try it yourself. Go to a physical space in which you feel comfortable about being overheard and chant words that have a long open vowel and a prolonged "Mmmmm" sound, such as the traditional chant of "Om" practiced for centuries by millions of Buddhist monks and their acolytes. Alternatively, you can opt for a simple "mmmm."

The more prolonged the sound you can make without stopping for breath, the more successful and quicker your results will be. Once more, do what you can. Ideally, you'll want to hold the note for at least 10 seconds; if that seems to you like a bridge too far, or a breath too far, don't worry about it. The key is to do it as best you can. If you're consistent, you'll find your ability to maintain that sound for longer and longer periods will quickly improve. If you can manage this practice for roughly ten minutes per session, you'll be well on your way to success. If you can perform three sessions every day, that's awesome. If once a day is all you can manage, then that's all you can manage. No one is going to chastise you and it is decidedly not a competition. Go for it, you high achiever, you! You'll feel a lot better a lot sooner in all likelihood because your vagus nerve will be able to recover quicker. Once again, do what you can and don't get down or give up because you're not able to achieve these goals immediately. It takes about three weeks to develop a consistent habit. Be patient with both these practices and yourself.

If you aren't noticing a quick return on these tactics on helping your mood, just hang in there. It will come with persistence. Keeping with the theme of practices traditionally associated with Asian cultures, the age-old practice of meditation increases vagal tone recovery, which, as we now understand, will subsequently spike our capacity for positive emotions as well the promotion of an increased sense of self-esteem according to extensive research. Now, a quick heads up for those who haven't practiced meditation before. The keyword is "practice." Even those who have practiced for a long time know that they will likely never achieve a state of nirvana, which, contrary to what many in the West believe is not synonymous with "heaven." The word actually comes from Sanskrit and means "nothingness."

The aim of meditation is to drain your mind of any thoughts other than existing in that exact moment. This is a worthy, albeit remarkably ambitious goal. Your concentration inevitably wanders at a speed and consistency that may shock you. It's hard to focus on a lack of focus. But just think of how much of your depression and anxiety you owe to worrying about the past and future. To experience a few seconds of relief from those temporal traps can be quite healing.

Make no mistake, meditation is by no means a "quick fix," but rather a practice that will not help with a quick return of your vagus nerve to top form. A long-term approach to its recovery and maintenance of a positive mindset is the key here. A regular, gentle regimen of meditation can often prove an excellent defense against relapses of those toxic emotional experiences.

For most people who suffer from depression and anxiety, even the periods in which those feelings ebb can't be enjoyed fully, as most sufferers are hyper vigilantly waiting for an omen that will help them see when anxiety or depression will come to assert itself once more.

Meditation also tends to increase your capacity to extend forgiveness and acceptance to yourself, which is an important life skill that many sufferers find especially difficult. Studies into this subject have also found that meditation reduces sympathetic "fight or flight" activity and increases vagal modulation.

As we know, the vagus nerve and the digestive system have a close, even intimate relationship. More than a few studies have shown the benefits of relaxation-related treatment for irritable bowel disorder (IBD). Want some more hard, pragmatic, scientific proof? A randomized controlled experiment of a relaxation-training intervention showed a demonstrable decrease in pain as well as decreased anxiety levels and improvements in quality of life. Anyone who suffers from IBD will have no trouble believing the latter assertion.

Conversely, another way of healing our vagal tone can yield relatively quick results. Is there a catch? Well, there always is, right? If there was a sure way to fix everything, we'd have already told you. Having said that, some of you will be fine with this technique and perhaps even enjoy it. For others, it can feel jarring. However, it is worth doing because of its benefits to the vagus nerve. This method is exposure to cold. We're not referring here to bitter, frostbite-inducing cold, but exposure to cold is never a welcome thought.

Acute exposure to cold (where acute is open to interpretation) activates the vagus nerve and its various neural pathways in a way that, if the vagus nerve were capable of feeling love, it would fall in love with it.

Another argument in favor of exposure to cold is that we now know that exposing yourself to cold on a regular basis can lower your sympathetic "fight or flight" responses as well as significantly tamper down the parasympathetic nerves. We've already seen that these nerves can sometimes all but overwhelm the vagus nerve if their activity is persistent to the point where the nerve itself becomes injured.

Remember the ice bucket craze from a few years back? You could try to bring that back. Or, perhaps more practically, when you've completed your shower, stand under the showerhead for at least 30 seconds while turning the tap to the coldest level you can stand. Eventually, you'll become acclimatized to it (at least a bit) and then you'll be able to increase your time under the cold water to 45 seconds, a minute, and even beyond. Your vagus nerve will find it invigorating and highly conducive to healing.

We've all heard the expression, "Laughter is the best medicine!" While not backed by science, even the grumpiest person can attest to feeling a lot better after laughing out loud. Talk to your funniest friends, binge on your favorite comedies, do whatever helps you smile and laugh when you feel down as often as you can. At first, you may not feel much in the mood for laughter; in fact, there's a strong chance you won't be. But you don't need to laugh for hours at a time to gain something from this.

The evidence for humor as an aid in emotional and even physical recovery has long been documented, but doctors weren't necessarily sure why this was the case. As it turns out, it's the vagus nerve (if you haven't been able to see that coming, well, spoiler: pretty much everything we're writing about here is going to, in one way or another, come back to that). Persistent laughter that does not have to be a belly laugh to be effective is very good for the vagus nerve. What you're aiming for here is consistently exposing yourself to situations (social and private) in which you are likely to find humor in something; this simple and enjoyable practice has been found to improve vagal tone, specifically through better rates of heart-rate variability.

Of course, a depressed or anxious person usually finds that laughter may not come easily or perhaps at all for a little while. But just as much as monitoring your heart rate, it's an easy and important way of charting any recovery you may be experiencing for yourself. Sometimes improvements lead to more improvements and that's what we're trying to achieve here.

And speaking of pleasant ways to help our vagus nerve, here's a rare advantage for those of you suffering from these ailments. You can guilt your partner or friend into a steady regimen of massage and, in particular, foot massage. Instead of it sounding like pampering, you can let your significant other know that you need them to give you a massage to help you feel better. Boom! You've got them! And you won't even be lying. The vagus nerve responds positively to the touch of others, and in particular, a massage. This is the best way to treat your low moods so you should grab it with both hands.

Another suggestion you likely weren't expecting to find in this book are coffee enemas. However, there are many people who speak of its proven invigorating properties. Which brave adventurer first thought to do this is lost to history, alas, but why it works makes perfect scientific sense. A key part of coffee's power is its caffeine content, which is effective in several ways. What it does in enema form is that it produces a reaction that both expands and moves the bowels (listen, we're not entirely thrilled to be going down this path, but it is science). The essential part of this procedure, in order to attain its maximum effect, is to resist the feeling you will experience to release your bowels. The longer you can resist, the more you can train your gut and, consequently, the vagus nerve, to move your bowels more consistently. You may, perhaps, be wondering what is the upside of this, medically speaking? The more consistently your bowels move, the more your body detoxifies itself. The benefits of this to your body are manifold. The vagus nerve has a role to play in even this seemingly routine but very important role.

We've saved gargling for last because we thought that you'd find it as strange to do to help your vagus nerve as we did. That is not a typo. Gargling actually makes sense, given how many muscles are connected with the vagus nerve. I bet you didn't see that coming. But it is completely true.

There's no need to explain to most readers of this book that many of the things that have usually given you pleasure, such as movies, music, sports, and even good food suddenly bring you no joy whatsoever. This condition is known as anhedonia. This word comes from ancient Greek and it means an inability to experience pleasure in virtually any form. If there's a better summation of the experience of deep depression, we've yet to hear it.

And as we've said so many times already, when you're feeling better, you're helping your vagus nerve get back into shape, which will in turn help you defeat anxiety and depression. Winston Churchill, along with Abraham Lincoln and a host of other politicians, suffered from chronic depression and termed this condition, "the black dog." Lincoln referred to it as "the noonday demon." John Lennon sang about it as the "blue mist round my soul." We lack their gift with language, so we'll opt for the more basic description. Depression is one of the worst experiences that a person can have to deal with in their life. That is why our relatively newfound understanding of the importance of the vagus nerve is such a promising development in the treatment of this crippling emotional disease.

Chapter 5

Other Treatments: The Ones Involving People in White Coats

So, just how new is this seeming treasure trove of information? Well, the discovery of the feedback loop we discussed earlier between the vagus nerve and our bodily symptoms of anxiety and depression has emerged in terms of methodically supervised studies within the last decade or so.

One approach that seems to hold some promise is known as craniosacral therapy. A CST is done by a very specific type of massaging rhythm aimed at easing the ready flow of cerebrospinal fluid in the area where the brain meets the spinal cord. According to the website Food For The Brain's article, "Vagus Nerve Function is The Missing Link to Improving Mental Health," a CST "practitioner will use their hands to feel for ease of motion and rhythm of cerebrospinal fluid surrounding the brain and spinal cord. They will then use soft-touch techniques (typically 5 grams about the weight of a nickel) to release restrictions in any tissues which surround the central nervous system."

This approach, some doctors and practitioners argue, will aid the vagus nerve. However, we should note that exactly how CST works is merely a matter of informed speculation among scientists, with many different theories currently circulating. There is also not a clear consensus that craniosacral therapy even does work. There are many different theories. What is largely agreed upon is that CST is very safe for the vast bulk of people, although people with conditions such as "acute aneurysm, cerebral hemorrhage, recent spinal cord or head injuries or severe bleeding disorders," should not attempt CST. CST is such a gentle, non-invasive treatment, it is even performed on infants. The rare side effects are not especially serious and are usually temporary. They include, according to www.hopeinstilled.org, "lightheadedness, dizziness, heavy sensation in head, nausea, or pain in the lower back." But it is worth keeping an eye out on the results of more and more CST studies, as research of treatments is accelerating our knowledge of the vagus nerve, and treatments continue to improve at a jaw-dropping speed.

Several studies focused on a transcutaneous treatment for a damaged vagus nerve. Transcutaneous just means under the skin, so it is similar to an injection. This type of vagus nerve stimulation (known as VNS to doctors) has shown conclusively that this type of therapy works at least as well as an earlier treatment, known technically as vagus nerve stimulation. VNS is an FDA-approved therapy that gives doctors another weapon against both depression and, oddly enough, epilepsy.

VNS, however, is a serious undertaking and is only allowed to be tried after several steps. It's for this reason that doctors are limited in their ability to employ this treatment. For one, they aren't allowed to use this therapy as a first resort.

Only after several different treatments are attempted with no effects on the patient's condition, a psychological state known technically as "treatment-resistant depression" is diagnosed. The patient undergoes a thorough physical examination to establish the patient's ability to withstand surgery and then doctors can attempt VNS. The procedure may seem like a superhero origin story, but it boils down to the surgeon implanting a device under the skin in the patient's chest that has the ability to consistently elevate the patient's mood.

According to an article published in a 2018 edition of Frontiers in Psychiatry magazine, a pilot study that examined the application of VNS in 60 patients with treatment-resistant depressive disorder showed a "significant clinical improvement in 30–37% of patients and a high tolerability." That number was large enough to give many psychologists and psychiatrists skepticism and optimism in equal measure.

To help disabuse many skeptics of their doubts, more tests were done, most of them confirming the treatment's great promise. Five years later, the stimulation of the vagus nerve for the treatment of "refractory depression" (essentially, another term for "treatment resistant depression") was approved by the U.S. Food and Drug Administration, which is not easy to do without an extended period of rigorous testing.

Certainly, VNS seems a very promising treatment, but it is not something you want to try until other methods have been exhausted. Nonetheless, more than 10,000 people have undergone the procedure over the last twelve years and it seems a logical assumption as this approach becomes both more refined and better known that these numbers will increase. Although the first iteration of this surgery often had unpleasant side effects (lower facial weakness being just one) these unfortunate occurrences have largely resolved themselves in recent years as the surgery has improved. For the vast majority of people, vagus nerve stimulation is safe. In January of 2022, a new generation of this vagal electrical stimulation (also known as neuromodulation) was developed into a smaller, singular neurotransmitter, which is currently tested on mice. This may lead to even smaller, more precise, and consistently reliable alternative therapies with fewer chances of side effects.

However, in rare cases, there are occasional side effects, most of them temporary. Temporary vocal cord paralysis is possible and so is permanent paralysis. Other side effects include hoarseness, swallowing difficulties, change in voice, persistent headaches, shortness of breath, persistent cough, and insomnia. If you suffer from sleep apnea, it may also exacerbate that.

We feel compelled to include the potential downsides of a VNS implant, but we also do not wish to overemphasize them, either. The list of ailments we listed in the previous paragraph are usually temporary and extremely rare. VNS is something worth talking to your clinician about. The FDA, as we stated earlier, has approved VNS procedures, but only if the patient meets the following criteria:

1. Has chronic, hard-to-treat depression (treatment-resistant depression).

2. Has failed to improve after a minimum of four medications and electroconvulsive therapy (ECT) or both.

3. Continues depression treatments in conjunction with vagus nerve stimulation.

In Europe, scientists in Antwerp, Belgium, began using VNS for the treatment of tinnitus (damage to hearing in which the sufferer hears a constant hum or buzz in their ears) after researchers at The University of Texas discovered that VNS was exceptionally good at softening or eliminating it. The results of this study were published in 2011, which may seem a long time ago. This is a small tick of the clock in terms of scientific knowledge that shows that our understanding of these procedures is yielding unforeseen benefits.

Oddly, scientists are not entirely sure why it works. Rest assured, they're working hard to figure that out. That's actually not as uncommon as you might think. We can take this revelation as a positive or negative thing. Scientists do know that it seems to work on many patients for whom there seemed to be little hope of ever escaping the long shadow of depression and anxiety.

We also do know that VNS alters the activity of many areas of the brain. The vagus nerve has structural connections with several mood-regulating limbic (part of the brain that regulates emotions) and cortical (the part of the brain that is largely responsible for our five primary senses) areas of the brain. PET scans consistently show declines in resting brain activity in the ventromedial prefrontal cortex that acts as the limbic system's immediate superior. VNS results in chemical changes in those parts of our brains, which goes a long way, perhaps, to explain its antidepressant effects. We gave a one-sentence summary of what VNS entails, but some of you may want a slightly deeper dive because we are, after all, talking about surgery.

In a VNS procedure, surgeons implant a device that will use mild electrical impulses in order to stimulate the vagus nerve. This stimulator is, again, FDA-approved to treat both depression and anxiety, as well as epilepsy. There's one vagus nerve on each side of your body, running from your brainstem through your neck to your chest and abdomen. When this VNS is activated, the device will send electrical signals along the vagus nerve to your brain stem, which in turn forwards these signals to certain areas in your brain. Doctors perform this operation on the left vagus nerve, as the right vagus nerve is more likely to affect the heart.

Surgery to implant the vagus nerve stimulation device is at times done on an outpatient basis, though there are many doctors who recommend an overnight hospital stay. The surgery itself usually takes between 60 and 90 minutes to complete, during which you may be given a localized anesthetic or a general one. If you are worried about the notion of any surgery that involves mucking around your brain, there's some good news for you, this surgery doesn't actually involve your brain. The surgeons will make two incisions, one on your chest or in your armpit and the other on the left side of the neck.

The surgeons then place what's known as the "pulse generator" in the upper left side of your chest. The device is meant to be a permanent addition to your body, but if there are persistently negative side effects, it can be removed. This device is roughly the size of a pocket watch and is powered by a battery. A wire is connected to the pulse generator. That wire is then connected to your vagus nerve.

The pulse generator will be turned on a few weeks later during a visit to your doctor. Afterward, its job is to deliver electrical impulses to the vagus nerve at varying currents and lengths of time. As a rule, vagus nerve stimulation usually begins at a very low level and then will gradually increase until it reaches an optimal level. According to the Mayo Clinic, "adjusting the electrical impulses can help minimize these effects. If side effects are intolerable, the device can be shut off temporarily or permanently".

The stimulator doesn't detect symptoms. Once activated, it will cycle on and off at intervals which will be decided upon by your doctor. You can use a specially devised magnet to temporarily turn off the vagus nerve stimulation, which may be necessary when you do certain activities such as public speaking, singing, or exercising, or when you're eating if you have swallowing problems. You'll visit your doctor on a regular basis, of course, to make sure that all systems are continuing to function optimally. But if VNS surgery doesn't sound like your cup of tea, the good news is that VNS surgery isn't the only medical treatment that can help with ailments involving the vagus nerve.

There is another treatment, known as tVNS, which is a non-invasive technique. This procedure centers on sending painless electrical currents to electrodes placed on specific areas on your body, most commonly targeting the vagus nerve, particularly the vagus nerve located in the neck. This technique, some doctors claim, elicits hypoactivation and hyperactivation in the sections of the brain that affect mood, which means the effects in the treatment of anxiety and depression, both long- and short-term, can be as harmful as they can be effective.

Nonetheless, this treatment seems to have yielded largely positive results in its first few years. The Wall Street Journal said of tVNS, "Columbia University Associate Clinical Professor of Psychiatry Richard P. Brown says he has used the device with 400 severely depressed patients and that more than 70% find relief -- about twice the rate of antidepressants that help regulate depression and anxiety."

The FDA, however, isn't quite as impressed as of now, and has yet to give its seal of approval to this newer, less-proven treatment. They're not alone in this. A study published in the December 2021 issue of "Science Direct" concluded that "It is uncertain whether tVNS reduces depressive symptoms and anxiety. Although existing studies show promising results, further studies are needed to increase the certainty of evidence." Conversely, the researchers admit that, "Available studies are few and heterogeneous, have major study limitations, problems with directness and imprecision."

This lack of hard and conclusive evidence hasn't stopped many companies from building their own versions of tVNS and peddling them online. Though some studies on tVNS treatment show clear promise, many other scientific inquiries have proven less than conclusive.

Nevertheless, some doctors, exasperated by the lack of progress of more traditional methods, can sometimes be persuaded to try it. These techniques have been approved in Europe to treat epilepsy, depression, and chronic pain. However, although they have yet to grant their approval, the FDA may soon get on board. According to the Mayo Clinic, some limited treatments have been given a preliminary permission, such as a "noninvasive device that stimulates the vagus nerve was recently approved by the Food and Drug Administration for the treatment of cluster headaches in the United States."

The fact that treating the vagus nerve can be used to cure or ameliorate various ailments is not only an exciting prospect for both patients and doctors but also another reason to feel optimistic that the FDA is looking at such treatments. For example, roughly one-third of those who suffer from epileptic seizures either don't respond or don't respond fully to anti-seizure drugs targeted for epilepsy. Vagus nerve stimulation, either via operation or non-invasive means, maybe an option to reduce the frequency of seizures in people who haven't achieved control of them with medications.

Additionally, researchers believe that such procedures may aid in the future treatment for a myriad of conditions, including persistent headaches, rheumatoid arthritis, bipolar disorder (again, a subset of the depressive category), IBS, and obesity. Some scientists also hope that these treatments may help to tackle Alzheimer's disease.

It can take months or longer after the procedure before you would notice any clear improvements in your depression or anxiety symptoms. Implanted vagus nerve stimulation isn't a panacea, but it seems to offer promise as another effective treatment in the battle against this disease.

Some of the latest and most important medical studies also indicate tVNS can help in not only treating these diseases, but can allow doctors to try to work preemptively to mitigate or prevent the disease before it has a real chance to catch hold. We now strongly believe that if a pregnant woman has a poor vagal tone during pregnancy, there is a fair chance that it will be passed down to her child.

Again, it is hard to overstate how new the notion of the vagus nerve as central to all manner of mental disorders as well as disorders of the brain really is. And while pessimists might lament that we don't know all we need to already, we would counsel these pessimists to have a little patience. Because the flow of new information about the vagus nerve comes almost too fast to keep track of, and the news frequently contains bombshell revelations.

For example, conclusive studies done in 2016 showed that stimulation of the vagus nerve could very well help reduce symptoms in not only the treatment of rheumatoid arthritis but other inflammatory diseases, such as Crohn's disease, Parkinson's disease, and Alzheimer's disease. Individuals who had previously failed to show any signs of improvement after other treatments consistently reported tangible and statistically marked improvements when they underwent treatments that centered on healing the vagus nerve, while, according to the online medical journal Medical News Today, not many "serious adverse side effects were noted."

CHAPTER 6

— · —

YOU ARE WHAT YOU EAT (QUITE LITERALLY, TO AN EXTENT)

We spoke earlier about how a good diet will help the vagus nerve. However, what do we mean by "good" in the context of the vagus nerve? Well, if you recall, we briefly mentioned probiotics, and while there are too many foods to list here (yogurt is a big one), we should perhaps take a moment to understand exactly what probiotics are. But first, a brief word in defense of an organism that has gotten a lot of bad press throughout the years, the misunderstood bacteria.

As you may know, our bodies are absolutely brimming with bacteria. What's the numerical equivalent of "brimming"? As it turns out, it's 39 trillion, give or take a few. Obviously, if our bodies have so much bacteria, they can't all be bad. In fact, not only are many of these bacteria not bad, but also quite a few are necessary to keep us alive. Studies performed on animals have shown strong evidence that certain bacteria are a key component of communication with the brain. Of course, this involves the vagus nerve, which oversees these communications. These benefits have a profound, positive impact on behavior and mood. So, how can we facilitate this improved communication involving the vagus nerve? By using probiotics.

Probiotics are vital in maintaining the health of good bacteria that is mostly found in our digestive systems. They help to stimulate the efficiency of acid that we will mercifully only refer to by its acronym, GABA. GABA is a neurotransmitter (something that transmits signals from the nerves to the brain). GABA has several functions and its presence has the effect of calming feelings of anxiety. When the vagus nerve receives probiotics, it produces larger quantities of GABA, which as we've just explained, is obviously an emotional and physical boon.

Again, animal experiments involving probiotics have been fairly conclusive in their health-promoting properties. As just one example, experiments have demonstrated, according to Frontiers in Psychiatry magazine, "that chronic treatment of mice with Lactobacillus Rhamnosus (a type of probiotic) caused a reduction in stress-induced corticosterone levels and in anxiety-like and depression-like behavior."

Even more glaring and promising in their conclusions are the experiments which have shown distinct differences in the composition of the bacteria in the digestive systems of patients with depression in contrast with those of healthy individuals. Further, biological samples pooled from five patients with depression transferred into mice without those bacteria have resulted in depressive-like behavior. The conclusion seems clear. The happier our guts and our vagus nerve, the happier our outlook on the world is.

Another mental health issue, namely, PTSD, seems to respond specifically well to probiotics. Indeed, probiotics may potentially decrease stress-induced anxieties such as PTSD. One exploratory experiment showed that patients diagnosed with PTSD and other trauma-related anxieties showed lower levels of probiotic bacteria in their digestive systems.

Probiotics do even more things to help the vagus nerve, such as enabling it to help stave off excessive inflammation, whose negative consequences we went into some depth about earlier. The bottom line is that it's in your best interests both physically and emotionally to eat a diet rich in probiotics. Before any changes to your diet, even if it is to add healthier choices, you should consult with your physician so they can counsel you on the best and safest choices to make that are tailored to you.

Let's talk about two words we generally don't associate with good health, namely, fatty acids. Our bodies need them. They really need them. Remember a while back when we described the human body as being not quite perfect? Well, Omega-3 acids would be a good example of why. Without a supply of Omega-3 acids, we would die. And yet our bodies cannot produce these fatty acids. They are acquired entirely through our diet. The omega-3 fatty acids present in seafood, for example, have a myriad of health benefits. Most of them are related to the health of the vagus nerve. They can help lower blood pressure (the vagus nerve is involved with the circulatory system), which of course means that they act as impediments to heart attacks, heart arrhythmia, and strokes.

If Omega-3 acids gave us those things and only those things, we would still prostrate ourselves in gratitude metaphorically. But Omega-3 acids are not only about these things. They play a key role in enhancing brain function as well as the development of vision and nerves for infants. Granted, newborns do not appreciate a well-prepared salmon, which is why nature has chosen to go the breast milk route as the best means to introduce Omega-3 acids into infants' systems.

Fish can make you smarter. Studies show that those who make fish a regular part of their diet have up to 14% larger hippocampus sections in their brains. The hippocampus houses most of our capacities for memory and learning. Fatty acids like Omega 3 are indispensable to our health and well-being.

Let's not misunderstand what we mean when we use the word "fatty." Some fat is good for us, while another fat is not. We're not saying you can't eat a cheeseburger or an ice-cream sundae on occasion; by all means, live a little. Just don't think you're doing any part of your body other than your taste buds any favors.

But there are such things as good fats, and the Omega-3 fats are at the top of that list. They are primarily found in fish (salmon is especially rich in them) as well as walnuts and seaweed. These specific fatty acids are essential for, among other things, the maintenance and improved function of the vagus nerve.

Tryptophan, an essential amino acid for humans and also, more famously, the reason you can barely keep awake after Thanksgiving dinner, is also a vital nutrient for maintaining a strong vagal tone. How, precisely, can something that makes us so sleepy and lethargic also boost our spirits? This is because one of the tryptophan's most critical qualities lies in its ability to act as a contributor to the release of serotonin. This is likely the reason that lower tryptophan levels have been consistently associated with wider and deeper levels of depression. A little over 90% of all serotonin synthesis occurs in our digestive tracts, which is yet one more reason to treat your gut the right way. In addition to turkey, asparagus is also a tryptophan-rich food. Olive oil, too, makes a great supplement for gut health.

Kefir and kombucha are also treats that are filled with vagus-healing nutrients. Leafy green vegetables such as spinach are chock full of vagus-enriching nutrients, as is poultry. In addition to the aforementioned tryptophan, poultry tends to be high in zinc, which the vagus nerve can't get enough of. For those of the vegetarian or vegan persuasion, do not despair: there are plenty of zinc-rich alternatives such as almonds and chickpeas. Zinc supplements are also available. In fact, while we are on the topic of supplements, there are many dietary supplements targeted specifically at retaining and improving your vagal tone.

Sometimes, of course, you are also what you do not eat. For example, the variability of our heart rates, as we discussed earlier, is one indicator of our vagal tone. Some scientists have argued that intermittent fasting or reducing your daily calorie consumption helps encourage optimal heart rate variability. If this is true, periodic intermittent fasting may help to stimulate the vagus nerve.

Frankly, one fact almost all medical authorities do agree on is that most of us have a caloric intake that could use some trimming down. This does not apply to all of us, and the road to many eating disorders is paved with an obsessive count of calories. If you do, or feel you might suffer from such a disorder, it is of the utmost importance that you seek out help from a medical professional or continue to follow the course one has charted for you. Adult males, according to the U.S. Department of Health, generally require between 2,000-3000 calories per day to maintain weight, while most adult females need around 1,600-2,400 calories. If you track your calories for a few days, you may be surprised at your daily intake.

If your caloric intake is significantly above this range over the course of several days, you may want to consider cutting back.

This usually necessitates cutting back on foods that are not great for us and the vagus nerve anyway, so even if fasting isn't conclusively good for our vagal tone, for many of us, cutting back on our consumption of calories will likely help vagal tone. And let's not forget probiotics, which are the most direct line to a healthy digestive system by providing your stomach and intestines with healthy and helpful bacteria. A lower caloric intake may not be a bad idea, either.

CHAPTER 7

— · —

WHERE SHOULD I GO TO FIND MY "VAGUS WHISPERER"?

S o, by now, if you're still reading, you're aware that virtually all of the leading mental health medical researchers believe that the vagus nerve and its health is directly and intimately involved in virtually all aspects of your health to one degree or another. Most specifically, it controls your emotional life. You have also learned about a variety of activities, some more surprising perhaps than others, to keep our vagus nerve in shape or to return it to health. We've also discussed in some detail the many ways in which your dietary choices affect your gut health, which for all intents and purposes is synonymous with your vagus nerve health.

We hope and believe that you will find this information and the techniques we outlined to be a big help in helping to battle your feelings of depression and/or anxiety. Indeed, we believe they can do more than help. We believe that it can make the critical difference many of us need now more than ever. One thing we have yet to meaningfully discuss, however, is among the most basic of questions regarding the vagus nerve: whom should we turn to when it comes to the need to assess the health and prescribe treatment for our vagus nerves? We recommend you schedule an appointment with your neurologist (if you do not have one ask your health provider for recommendations).

As the vagus nerve is a neurological issue, your neurologist is your obvious first stop. However, although all neurologists are versed on vagal tone, it's still a very new field. Because of that, you'll want to make sure your doctor is an active proponent of the possibilities of vagal nerve treatment. Like any other medical theory in any other branch of medicine, there is a spectrum of knowledge and or enthusiasm for certain approaches and treatments, depending on the practitioner.

In fact, there are some doctors who have begun to concentrate the majority of their practices on the vagus nerve and its health. Again, such doctors should be reasonably easy to find and there are many such doctors in private practices, as well. Indeed, certain groups of doctors have established clinics, both virtually and in real life, that cater exclusively to patients and their vagal tones. Some of these groups are for-profit organizations, and while this by no means suggests they aren't staffed with brilliant and compassionate doctors, or as one such organization terms themselves, "polyvagalists," it is simply better to be aware of their status.

The bottom line is to do your research and not to be afraid, as much as your geographical and financial situations will allow you, to search for a while to find a doctor or team you feel will be most likely to address your needs. Treat it like buying a new car. You should probably be willing to be at least as exhaustive when it comes to searching for what your gut literally and figuratively tells you will best attend to your emotional peace of mind.

At the very beginning of this book, we spoke about the fact that depression and anxiety diagnoses have seen a steady upward curve during the last twenty years. We alluded to a couple of reasons behind this situation. But we didn't want to do a deep dive at that point, because we could almost hear you shouting "Get to the vagus nerve!" However, we want to explore this a little more in-depth. We certainly don't claim to have the answer to this multi-layered problem. The seeds of depression have not only bloomed but have also become overgrown. It does not seem like the issue is likely to go away any time soon either. From an evolutionary standpoint, society has transformed from living in small communities, where everyone knew each other all their lives and seldom traveled more than a few miles from their homes. We're not advocating we return to these days, but it's quite a radical departure from how we live today. Our bodies, including our vagus nerves, are having a hard time navigating cultural waters that have simply not been made for swimming in.

Here's another thing. Many of us, via social media, have come to have many of our interactions with others not in person. There are many interactions with people we've never met. Until very recently, most of us lived and interacted with only those we knew and only in person. So, what's the point? The point is that modern life has stripped most of us of a sense of context about others and, most critically, of ourselves. And this is innately disorienting, which sends panic signals to the vagus nerve, making it desperate to interpret an influx of data it doesn't have a firm enough footing to interpret. Just as we know context is important in a conversation in order to fully understand what's discussed, a viable and reliable context in which to interpret ourselves without any context of who we really are is critical to figure out who we are, both to ourselves and others. That's a sure-fire recipe for alienation. Alienation causes depression and anxiety as a natural reaction.

News channels spin rather than report, which by definition requires removing context from every story they report. Social media has a way of showing nothing but happiness and success to project to the world. Unless we know these people in real life, we can't really get to the truth of their lives (I originally typed "lies"' there. A Freudian typo). Even that goal is purely aspirational. The names of these social media sites, as we know, are Old Norse words meaning "Where nuance goes to die".

Faced with all of these forces, and with either a plethora of free time or not a minute to stop and breathe and evaluate, we are robbed of any real context of ourselves. The way we live our lives now strips us of the thing we used to be conscious of. Without context, you're looking at yourself in a funhouse mirror and you're also looking at the whole world that way. This has happened over a long period of time so we've failed to notice. We're not saying that's the whole answer by any stretch. We're just wondering if it isn't at least a part of it.

All of this is to say, self-blame is part of the dark ghosts that further cloud the minds of sufferers of the sometimes crippling effects of depression and anxiety. And if you walk away with one lesson from this book, then we've done a bad job. One of the key lessons we hope you come away with that is not directly related to the vagus nerve, its functions, and how to best maintain a healthy vagal tone, is that your illness is in no way a sign of weakness or "lack of character." There isn't a single sufferer who hasn't heard this more than once, often from people that we love. And they're just utterly, unambiguously wrong. In fact, given the world as it is these days, one can argue that feeling depressed is a sign of empathy and awareness. Not that this should ever stop you from trying to get better. Indeed, it should be a spur, because the world needs all the empathetic people it can get these days.

Some more promising news that is almost as important as the exciting frontiers being constantly discovered about the vagus nerve is the fact that in many corners of our society, depression, and anxiety are losing their stigma as a sign of weakness. Speaking candidly about it to others helps to educate people more but you are under zero obligation to ever do so. Your main priority is getting and staying well. And if that includes maintaining your privacy, 1) that's what you need to do and 2) taking care of yourself is at times a struggle in and of itself. Don't feel the obligation to educate others, as well. Some people find it helpful to talk about depression but many do not, and there's nothing wrong with either approach.

One thing that you might think about sharing is the miracle that is the vagus nerve because, as we hope this book has demonstrated, everyone benefits when their vagal tone is strong.

CHAPTER 8

—·—

POP QUIZ!

Remember when we promised you that there wouldn't be any quizzes? Well, that was sort of true. The good news is that there won't be any quizzes for you, but we are going to be put to the test (or quiz) by having your (or rather, our idealized sense of you) ask us the kind of questions we have thought you might ask. Sounds fun? Not to us, either, but let's face it, what else have you got going on right now? Exactly.

So, here are the rules: you (our rather, us, trying to channel you) will ask us questions about some of the many things we've discussed in this book which, sadly, is starting to wind down. Then we will do our best to answer "your" questions in a way that will reinforce what we've learned. Questions? Good. Okay, here we go:

True or false: depression and anxiety cause the economy of the United States to lose billions of dollars each year.

Answer: Absolutely. In fact, it is the single most common reason people call in sick to work (although they seldom admit this to their bosses, studies have shown).

· · · · ●· ●· · ·

True or false: Depression and Anxiety affect the vagus nerve, and vice-versa.

Answer: Nothing personal, but these questions are real softballs. We're worried you think we can't handle the tough stuff. After all, we wrote a book about it. Well, we almost have. We will very soon. As you can tell by holding it or looking at your e-reader, we're almost through. Anyway, the answer is a yes, yes, a thousand times yes! That, after all, is sort of the central point of this book. Our vagus system, for all of its remarkable abilities, is not terribly adept at proportionate responses. It is still thinking we're one step away from being eaten by a hungry wolf, when in fact we simply have an essay due next week or we haven't gotten a text back after 10 minutes from the person we've been on two dates with and. Sometimes, there's no reason at all or, at least, no reason that you can consciously discern.

· · · · ●· ●· · ·

Question: Of the seemingly endless parts of the body the vagus nerve plays a central role in, which one would you consider the most important?

Answer: Hmm, this is a trick question, isn't it? Well played, you, or us, or us as you, whatever. That's hard to say: so many are vital. It's like asking us to pick our favorite child. What we will say is that for the purposes of this book, the gut-brain connection is by far the most relevant when it comes to affecting anxiety and depression. We're going to cheat a little bit on this question by giving you a broad answer, and that is, the vagus nerve's most important function affects the issues of depression and anxiety. And it does so based on its relationship with controlling and monitoring our sympathetic nervous system.

For those of you who may have forgotten what the sympathetic nervous system does, and are frankly too lazy to go back to the beginning of the book (no judgment, here; in fact, in an odd way we have a lot of respect for that self-knowledge), it relays signals to the vagus nerve regarding the classic "fight or flight" mechanism. Some of you may be saying, "But I thought the adrenal gland handles that?" Yes, but what do you think gives the signal to the adrenal gland to get fired up? It is the sympathetic nervous system, acting on direct orders from the vagus nerve.

· · · · ● · ● · · ·

Question: What sort of foods should I eat in order to promote a strong vagal tone?

Answer: First of all, way to do a humble brag is by using the phrase "vagal tone." Foods rich in Omega-3 oils will work wonders for your vagal tone, and frankly, the rest of your mental and physical health. We provided a partial list of foods typically rich in these oils (remember, Omega-3 is vital to our health, but our bodies are incapable of producing it). Fish is the most common source but, as we saw earlier in the book, there are many other ways to get your share of Omega-3 acids as well. Tryptophan is also highly important in promoting good gut health and helping the vagus nerve.

· · · · ● · ● · · ·

Question: Are things such as mindfulness, deep breathing, and even yoga truly helpful in reducing our levels of stress?

Answer: Once more, the answer here is an unequivocal yes. All of these will help you to slow your breathing, clear your minds, and as a result, reassure the vagus nerve that all is well. Should you wear yoga pants outside of a yoga class setting? We don't feel qualified to answer. That question is best taken up with your partner or the context (for example, not on a job interview. Unless you're interviewing to be a yoga instructor).

· · · ● ● · ● ● · ·

Question: Will having a healthy vagus nerve solve all of our personal issues?

Answer: Umm, no. If there were a single thing that could do that and if we had knowledge of it, trust us, we would charge a lot more for this book. But what a healthy vagal tone will be able to help you with is coping with whatever you're going through, which, in a way, is perhaps even better. Challenges, as we all know, are very often good for us. They allow us to learn, grow as people, and accrue wisdom. But when we face life's challenges and become too overwhelmed or sometimes even feel overwhelmed by the simple act of being awake, our vagus nerve can play an important role in helping us to feel that we can grab hold of the reins of our lives once more. And that, we think we can all agree, is a skill well worth developing.

CHAPTER 9

—·—

DON'T THINK OF THIS AS GOODBYE, BUT RATHER AS A CHANCE TO CATCH UP ON OTHER BOOKS

We certainly hope we've been able to provide you with not only a sufficient amount of evidence to not only believe in the now irrefutable science that has taught us of the importance of the vagus nerve for our mental health, but also to embrace this fact as a clear and deeply helpful aid in coping with depression and anxiety. We also firmly believe we have provided you with sound strategies to help your vagus nerve help you.

It is odd to contemplate that something like depression, which, when it hits us, feels so deeply personal, so intrinsically linked, or even tightly woven into what many of us perceive as our most basic essence. This is what some may call the "soul," or for the less spiritually inclined, our true nature. For many, these feelings have been so pervasive, so powerful, and so constant and innate that it's easy to confuse them with the basic core of who we are.

Given our feelings, and our strange yet natural emotional attachment to these feelings, it's almost impossible for us to conceive of anything capable of untangling those feelings from our sense of self. And yet, the fact that you've got this book is proof that you're still willing to try. To do so is a risk and a real act of courage. If nothing else, you should take some pride in that fact and should not, as you may instinctively do, downplay it as a real show of character and strength.

And as odd a sense as the above can be, it is perhaps odder still that a nerve in our bodies can play such a large role in dictating our emotions. After all, what feels more intimate, inextricably you, than your emotions and internal lives? Some of you might even resent this notion. Some might find it somehow robs of our emotional autonomy.

We hear you; such feelings are natural. But what we want to emphasize is that our knowledge of the vagus nerve and how it can affect our emotions does not mean that it controls who you are any more than a lack of sleep nullifies your basic nature. Sure, you may be irritable or sleepy as a result, but you hardly make value judgments about who is at your core because of a bad night's sleep.

We hope you will view this information as an effective tool to reclaim who you truly are and give you a path to achieve all of your potential. Our understanding of mental health is still relatively new and our cultural attitudes towards it are even less enlightened. Don't let either of these circumstances prevent you from forging ahead to beat this illness and doing everything you can to defeat it. Unfortunately, we cannot give you a specific plan for how you should go about this specifically. We don't know you (although, in a sense, we like to think we've bonded during the course of this), so such decisions are obviously left to your healthcare provider. If you don't have a professional working with you on your emotional well-being, we urge in the strongest personal terms to get on that as soon as possible.

What we do feel confident in asserting, though, is that the health and maintenance of your vagus nerve will absolutely help you on the path to seeing the world through the clear lens you deserve. A lens without the dense fog of depression and anxiety. We feel confident that what you've learned here can be an invaluable tool in that quest.

And a quest is what it is and for many of us, it is a lifelong quest. We have every faith that you will succeed at this quest. We believe and know that we have provided you with a valuable weapon for this quest. We would wish you luck, but we have the utmost faith that with persistence, determination, and the right help (seeking out help is also not a sign of weakness or a failure of character any more than going to a surgeon when you need your tonsils removed), you will prevail.

We hope and believe you'll allow what we've learned here to be a part of your healing.

Milton Keynes UK
Ingram Content Group UK Ltd.
UKHW011603280723
425965UK00004B/171